Hudson Press

Recipes, Meal Plans, Tips & Tricks!

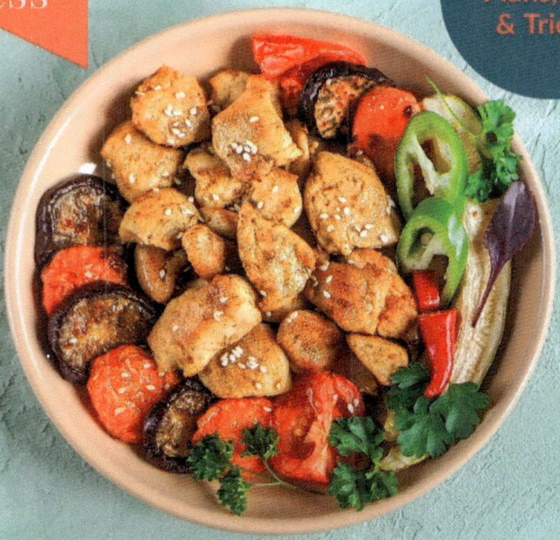

Diabetes Cookbook
& Meal Plan

Aqsa Layla, MD

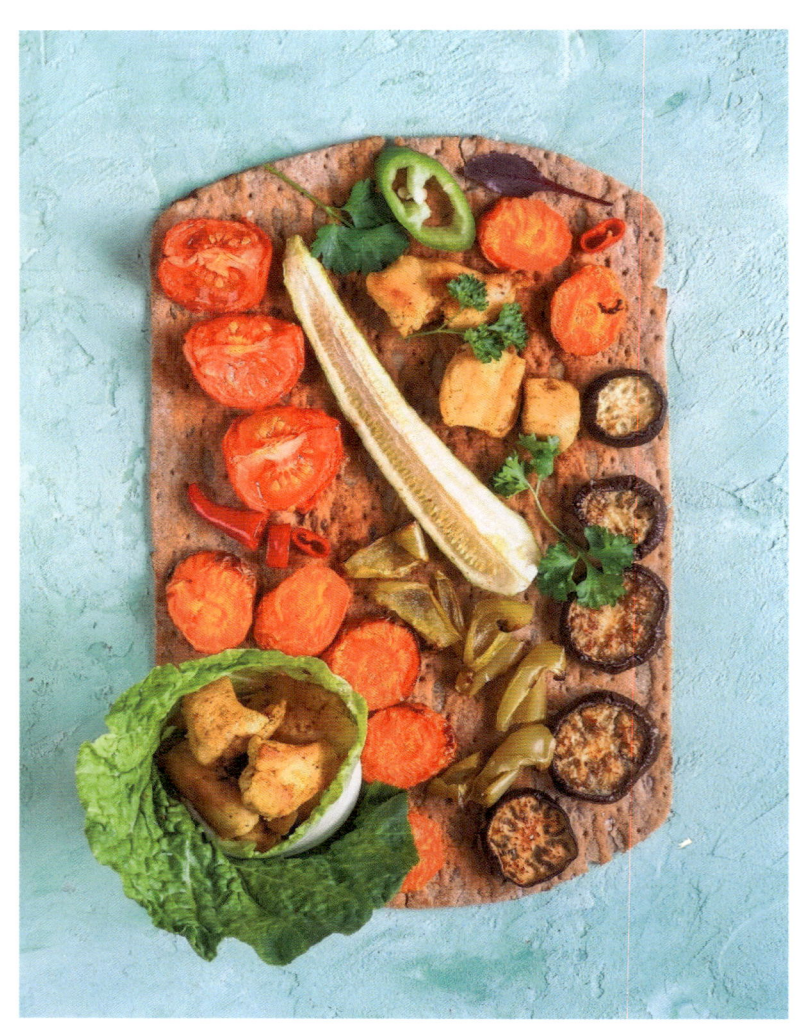

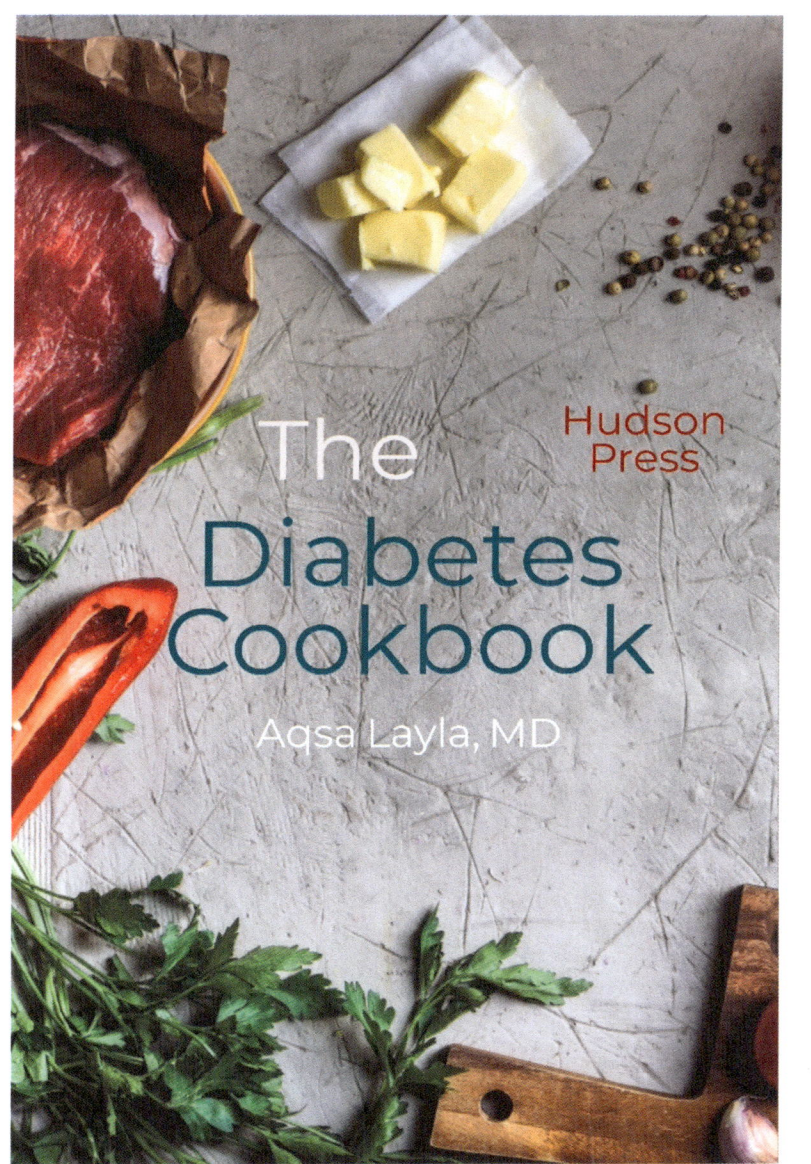

Contents

Introduction pg. 3

What is Diabetes? pg. 4-8

Causes of Diabetes pg.8-11

Types of Diabetes pg.12-14

Diabetic Diet pg.15-31

The Meal Plan pg. 33-37

Breakfast Recipe pg.38

Bacon Wrapped Egg Muffins pg.38-40

Blueberry Oat Pancakes pg.41-42

Salmon Cheese Wraps pg. 42-44

Hazelnut Cheese Breakfast pg. 44-45

Spinach Morning Muffins pg.45-47

Coco Protein Oats pg.47-48

Pumpkin Cinnamon Pancakes pg.49-50

Cauliflower Meal pg.50-51

Cheese Oats Pancakes pg.52-53

Bacon Bok Choy pg.53-54

Lunch Recipes pg.55

Roasted Cauliflower pg.55-56

Green Beans with Mushroom Sauce pg.56-58

Oysters with Almond Butter pg.59-60

Roasted Turnips pg.61-62

Escarole Cream Salad pg.62-64

Balsamic Tomato Chicken 64-66

Green Ham Soup pg.66-69

Chicken Cauliflower Casserole 69-71

Steak with Caramelized Fennel pg.71-72

Chicken Pesto Casserole pg.73-74

Dinner Recipes pg.75

Zucchini Mushroom Lasagna pg.75-77
Spinach Cheese Rolls pg.78-80
White Chicken Soup pg.80-82
Balsamic Turkey Breast pg.82-84
Avocado Beef Fajitas pg.84-86
Prosciutto Chicken pg.86-87
Pork Chops in Tomato Gravy pg.87-89
Queso Chicken Chili pg.89-91
Turkey Spinach Meatballs pg.92-93
Chicken Piccata pg.94-96

Dessert Recipes pg.97

Buckwheat Chocolate Cake pg.97-99
Meringue Custard Dessert pg.97-99
Avocado Brownies pg.99-101
Lemon Curd Pie pg.101-103
Peanut Butter Chocolate Brownie pg.105-106
Roasted Cashew Cookies pg.106-108
Creamy Chocolate Mousse pg.108-109
Coconut Bounty Bars pg.109-111
Blueberry Almond Tart pg.111-113
Chia Coco Pudding pg.113-115
07 Days Meal Plan pg.115-117
Conclusion pg. 118

Introduction

Time has brought us to the age of complexities, where nothing is simple to deal with. Unfortunately, health disorders top this list, as people are inflicted with various problems which are not completely curable and persistently affects their lives. Diabetes is one such health issue, which does not only restrict you from taking sugars, but can lead to other problems as well if not controlled or checked properly. There are cases of people suffering from diabetes living a normal life whereas others have their lives at risk due to the harms of this diseases. That is why it is vital to learn about the disease and the ways to contain it and possibly reverse it. An incurable disease it was once thought to be. However, recent data has proven otherwise. Less dependent on medicinal therapies and more dependent on a passive means of treatment, i.e., dietary therapy. Good food is no less than medicine, with the right dietary approach we can indeed control diabetes and even reverse diabetes in an effective manner. And that is the aim of this cookbook; we have created a complete diet plan for all the diabetic patients, to provide them both health and delight in a single platter.

What is Diabetes?

Diabetes is a hormonal disorder, which results in high blood glucose levels. Glucose is the driving fuel of our body. Everything we eat is finally broken down into glucose which is utilized by the cells to gain energy. This glucose is supplied to the body's organs through our blood. The excess is either discarded or stored in the body in some other forms. There has to be a certain balance of blood glucose to facilitate its better use. If the glucose level is too high, it can lead to numbness or even retardation. Or if too low, it can lead to hypoglycemia. This balance of glucose is maintained through two hormones namely Insulin and Glucagon. Glycogen allows the glucose to be released into the blood whereas Insulin does the opposite, i.e., a decrease in the blood glucose levels. In diabetes, the pancreatic cells producing the Insulin hormone are affected, and they reduce the Insulin production. This leads to the increase of glucose in the blood to a harmful level.

Ideally, a person should have 70 to 130 mg/dL glucose in the blood. If the amount increases and persists in the high range, the person will then be suffering from diabetes. Once the beta cells in the pancreas are damaged, they don't get to repair easily. That is why diabetes must be controlled, and then reversed.

Symptoms of Diabetes:

It is always important to detect the presence of disease at early stages to avoid maximum damage. Same is true for diabetes, far before going to a doctor, the following symptoms can be easily detected at home.

- **Constant Thirst**

This symptom is somehow related to the next one. Frequent loss of salt and water from the body can cause increased thirst. And this thirst cannot be quenched with more water, as your body will be losing in eventually. It can be dealt with only by dealing with diabetes in a better way.

- **Increased Urination:**

A surge in blood glucose level affects the working of the kidneys and them over function to cause more urination than normal. This urination is not healthy as it makes the patient loss lots of water and salts out of the body. It is the unwanted removal of the essential mineral from the body. So frequent urination should be taken seriously in any case. Else it will render the patient dehydrated.

- **Abrupt weight loss:**

Weight loss is the common symptom among patients of diabetes. They drastically lose several pounds if they are not on any sort of treatment. The excess of glucose makes the body to metabolize excessively or more than the extent needed. Eventually, the body fails to absorb nutrients for its building process, and the muscles lose their energy and weight. Same happens with the bones and other organs.

- **Affected Vision**

The sugar spike instantly affects the vision by mingling with the optic nerves in the brain and weakening the eye muscles or affecting the lens or the retina. If you witness a sudden vision change, then consult a doctor. Carelessness can even cause impairment in extreme cases.

- **Sudden Hunger**

The imbalance also causes hypoglycemia, which is the state of extreme hunger. This because of the fact that the body is incapable of harnessing the energy out of the food. It keeps the energy deficit and produces the sensation of extreme hunger. For this problem to deal, it is suggested to take a small amount of meal after every 1 to 2 hours.

- **Tiredness and Fatigue**

Fatigue is related to many chronic health disorders. It is also common among diabetic patients. They pretty much same the exhaustion all the time, even after rest. Get yourself check if that is the case.

- **Numbness of limbs**

The sensation in the hands and feet is great lost when you are suffering from diabetes. This is the reason many diabetic patients don't even feel pain in most parts of the body when hurt. This numbness can get into the way of the normal function of the hands and feet.

- **No Healing**

With diabetes, the body loses the normal function of healing. And it takes a longer duration of time to heal a sore or a wound. The infection may get serious if not treated properly in time. Use of additional medicines is prescribed for quick recovery.

Nausea, stomach pain, and vomiting are few of the additional symptoms which a patient may experience in the early or later stages of diabetes.

Causes of Diabetes

When we think of diabetes, many people blame sugars as the real enemy. That is not even close to reality. It is true that it may aggravate the harms of this condition, but it is not the cause of diabetes. The real causes are many, and any of these can lead to diabetes.

- **Resistance to Insulin**

The first possibility of having diabetes is the body's inability to react to the insulin. In this case, the pancreatic cells produce the insulin in a normal way, but this insulin is of no use as the body will not respond to it, and the blood glucose levels will not be managed. This condition is also termed as the 'prediabetes' because the glucose levels in this condition are not as high as in other diabetes, but they are not low enough to be considered as 'NO diabetes.'

- **Lack of insulin**

This is the primary cause of diabetes, where our pancreatic cells fail to produce sufficient insulin. In this case, there is not enough insulin to reverse the effects of glucagon in the body. Consequently, the glucose levels spike up. This condition can cause type II diabetes which is quite common among the people of old ages.

- **Genetic History**

Genes control every function of our body. Diabetes is not always caused by damage to the pancreas, but at times it can also be the result of genetic tendencies. According to the experts, a number of genetic disorders are also associated with insulin resistance or low production of insulin. That is why we see people belonging to a certain lineage suffering from diabetes than the others. Cystic fibrosis and hemochromatosis are two different conditions that damage the pancreas and leads to diabetes. Gene mutation can also be the reason for diabetes.

- **Obesity**

Stored fats and more weight can make the body more resistive towards insulin. When fatty acids are stored in the body, they may cause inflammation over pancreas or other parts of the body. This process can disrupt the functioning of insulin in the body. However, more research is now being conducted to link the relationship between diabetes and obesity to understand the cause more clearly.

- **Poor diet**

Poor diet can lead to a number of health problems, and diabetes is just one of them. It can increase the risks of contracting diabetes. Any diet low in minerals, fibers, vitamins and high in fats and carbohydrates can increase the risk of diabetes. It can either cause it through obesity or directly affecting the function of the pancreas.

Types of diabetes

Just as the causes of diabetes greatly vary, its types also vary, and each type is treated and controlled differently. If the cause is insulin resistance, you can not treat it by injecting more insulin. For that, you would need some other measures. So it is essential to know which type of diabetes you are suffering from. Here are the three types of diabetes:

1. **Type I:**

This type of diabetes is the result of the body's own autoimmune response. It means that our defense mechanism damages the pancreatic cells that produce insulin. As a result, our pancreas stops producing insulin or start producing them in an insufficient amount. This type of diabetes can happen at any time of your age, irrespective of your gender and the gene type. People suffering from diabetes type I need insulin to be injected artificially on day to day basis in order to maintain levels of glucose in their blood. They also can take insulin orally, but that it is usually not as effective as the direct injections.

2.   Type II:

90% of diabetic patients suffer from this type of diabetes. It is mostly diagnosed in people of adults ages, but today, young adults are also equally susceptible to the disease. This type of diabetes can stay undetected for several years as it can only be identified through special tests. Good diet and constant exercise can only control the harms of this diabetes. The patient may require some extra dose of insulin both orally or through injections. It is also known as the 'Prediabetes,' and it is caused due to the inability of the body to respond to the insulin production in the body. There is no apparent damage to the cells producing the insulin unlike type I diabetes.

3.   Gestational diabetes (GDM)

As the name indicates it, this type of diabetes can occur to a mother during the gestational period or pregnancy. The good news is that it is not permanent but a temporary condition and persists only during the pregnancy. It is caused by the production of certain hormones from the placenta of the baby, and these hormones can disrupt the functioning of the insulin. So the body becomes insulin resistant. It is not always harmful, but the condition can get critical in case of malnutrition or poor dietary intake.

Diabetic Diet

Treatment through dietary approach is considered most effective and logical today. Many of the fatal health conditions are now treated only with a well-oriented health diet plan. Same is true for diabetes. With few adjustments in the routine menu, a patient can maintain his glucose levels without the use of medicines. To make this idea to work, we need to cut down the direct or high sources of glucose in the food. Here is the complete list of the items which can be taken on a diabetes-friendly diet.

What to Have on a Diabetic Diet:

- **Vegetables:**

Fresh vegetables never cause harm to anyone. So adding a meal full of vegetables is the best shot for all diabetic patients. But not all vegetables contain the same amount of macronutrient. Some vegetables contain a high amount of carbohydrates, so those are not suitable for a diabetic diet. We need to use the vegetables which contain a low amount of carbohydrates.

1. Cauliflower

2. Spinach
3. Tomatoes
4. Broccoli
5. Lemons
6. Artichoke
7. Garlic
8. Asparagus
9. Spring onions
10. Onions
11. Ginger etc.

- **Meat:**

Meat is not on the red list for the diabetic diet. It is fine to have some meat every now and then for diabetic patients. However certain meat types are better than others. For instance, red meat is not a preferable option for such patients. They should consume white meat more often whether its seafood or poultry. Healthy options in meat are:

1. All fish, i.e., salmon, halibut, trout, cod, sardine, etc.
2. Scallops

3. Mussels

4. Shrimp

5. Oysters etc.

- **Fruits:**

Not all fruits are good for diabetes. To know if the fruit is suitable for this diet, it is important to note its sugar content. Some fruits contain a high amount of sugars in the form of sucrose and fructose, and those should be readily avoided. Here is the list of popularly used fruits which can be taken on the diabetic diet:

1. Peaches
2. Nectarines
3. Avocados
4. Apples
5. Berries
6. Grapefruit
7. Kiwi Fruit
8. Bananas
9. Cherries
10. Grapes
11. Orange

12. Pears
13. Plums
14. Strawberries

- **Nuts and Seeds:**

Nuts and seeds are perhaps the most enriched edibles, and they contain such a mix of macronutrients which can never harm anyone. So diabetic patients can take the nuts and seeds in their diet without any fear of glucose spike.

1. Pistachios
2. Sunflower seeds
3. Walnuts
4. Peanuts
5. Pecans
6. Pumpkin seeds
7. Almonds
8. Sesame seeds etc.

- **Grains:**

Diabetic patients should also be selective while choosing the right grains for their diet. the idea is to keep the amount of starch as minimum as possible. That is why you won't any see any white rice in the list rather it is replaced with more fibrous brown rice.

1. Quinoa
2. Oats
3. Multigrain
4. Whole grains
5. Brown rice
6. Millet
7. Barley
8. Sorghum
9. Tapioca

- **Fats:**

Fat intake is the most debated topic as far as the diabetic diet is concerned. As there are diets like ketogenic, which are loaded with fats and still proved effective for the diabetic patient. The key is the absence of carbohydrates. In any other situation, the fats are as harmful to diabetics than any normal person. Switching to unsaturated fats is a better option.

1. Sesame oil
2. Olive oil
3. Canola oil
4. Grapeseed oil
5. Other vegetable oils
6. Fats extracted from plant sources.

- **Diary:**

Any dairy product which directly or indirectly causes a glucose rise in the blood should not be taken on this diet. other than those, all products are good to use. These items include:

1. Skimmed milk
2. Low-fat cheese
3. Eggs
4. Yogurt
5. Trans fat-free margarine or butter

- **Sugar Alternatives:**

Since ordinary sugars or sweeteners are strictly forbidden on a diabetic diet. There are artificial varieties which can add sweetness without raising the level of carbohydrates in the meal. These substitutes are:

1. Stevia
2. Xylitol
3. Natvia
4. Swerve
5. Monk fruit
6. Erythritol

Make sure to substitute them with extra care. The sweetness of each sweetener is entirely different from the table sugar, so add each in accordance with the intensity of their flavor. Stevia is the sweetest of them, and it should be used with more care. In place of 1 cup of sugar, a teaspoon of stevia is enough. All other sweeteners are more or less similar to sugar in their intensity of sweetness.

Foods to avoid

Knowing a general scheme of diet helps a lot, but it is equally important to be well familiar with the items which have to be avoided. With this list, you can make your diet a hundred percent sugar-free. There are many other food items which can cause some harm to a diabetic patient as the sugars do. So let's discuss them in some detail here.

- **Sugars:**

Sugar is a big NO GO for a diabetic diet. Once you are diabetic, you would need to say goodbye to all the natural sweeteners which are loaded with carbohydrates. They contain polysaccharides which readily breaks into glucose after getting into our body. And the list does not only include table sugars but other items like honey and molasses should also be avoided.

1. White sugar
2. Brown sugar
3. Confectionary sugar
4. Honey
5. Molasses
6. Granulated sugar

It is not easy to sudden stop using sugar. Your mind and your body, both will not accept the abrupt change. It is therefore important to go for a gradual change. It means start substituting it with low carb substitutes in a small amount, day by day.

- **High Fat Dairy Products:**

Once you are diabetic, you may get susceptible to a number of other fatal diseases including cardiovascular once. That is why experts strictly recommend avoiding high-fat food products especially the dairy items. The high amount of fat can make your body insulin resistance. So even when you take insulin, it won't be of any use as the body will not work on it.

- **Saturate Animal Fats:**

Saturated animal fats are not good for anyone, whether diabetic or normal. So, better avoid using them in general. Whenever you are cooking meat, try to trim off all the excess fat. Cooking oils made out of these saturated fats should be avoided. Keep yourself away from any of the animal origin fats.

- **High Carb Vegetables:**

As discussed above, vegetables with more starch are not suitable for diabetes. These veggies can increase the carbohydrate levels of the food. So omit these from the recipes and enjoy rest of the less starchy vegetables. Some of the high carb vegetables are:

1. Potatoes
2. Sweet potatoes
3. Yams etc.

- **Cholesterol Rich ingredients:**

Bad cholesterol or High-density Lipoprotein has the tendency to deposit in different parts of the body and obstructs the flow of blood and the regulation of hormones. That is why food items having high bad cholesterol are not good for diabetes. Such items should be replaced with the ones with low cholesterol.

- **High Sodium Products:**

Sodium is related to hypertension and blood pressure. Since diabetes is already the result of a hormonal imbalance in the body, in the presence of excess sodium another imbalance- the fluid imbalance may occur which a diabetic body cannot tolerate. It adds up to already present complications of the disease. So, avoid using food items with a high amount of sodium. Mainly store packed items, processed foods and salt all contain sodium, and one should avoid them all. Use only the 'Unsalted' variety of food products, whether its butter, margarine, nuts or other items.

- **Sugary Drinks:**

Cola drinks or other similar beverage are filled with sugars. If you had seen different video presentations showing the amount of the sugars present in a single bottle of soda, you would know how dangerous those are for diabetic patients. They can drastically increase the amount of blood glucose level within 30 minutes of drinking. Fortunately, there are many sugar-free varieties available in the drinks which are suitable for diabetic patients

- **Sugar Syrups and Toppings:**

A number of syrups available in the markets are made out of nothing but sugar. Maple syrup is one good example. For a diabetic diet, the patient should avoid such sugary syrups and also stay away from the sugar-rich toppings available in the stores. If you want to use them at all, trust yourself and prepare them at home with a sugar-free recipe.

- **Sweet Chocolate and candies:**

For diabetic patients, sugar-free chocolates or candies are the best way out. Other processed chocolate bars and candies are extremely damaging to their health, and all of these should be avoided. You can try and prepare healthy bars and candies at home with sugar-free recipes.

- **Alcohol:**

Alcohol has the tendency to reduce the rate of our metabolism and take away our appetite, which can render a diabetic patient into a very life-threatening condition. Alcohol in a very small amount cannot harm the patient, but the regular or constant intake of alcohol is bad for health and glucose levels.

Glycemic index and Diabetes:

It is a scale which was created to rate the food items in accordance with the number of carbohydrates present in them. It has set the standard value to compare and identify the glucose level in a food item.it has given a 100 score to glucose Itself. This value is taken as a standard, and all other items are compared with this value and ranked accordingly. Anything having an equal amount of carbs as the glucose will have the glycemic index value 100. Any food item having half of the carbs than glucose will show the GI value of 50. So, this index is basically referential, and it is the result of the comparison.

GI value is also representative of the blood sugar levels of a person. It is calculated as the effect of the food taken. After about two hours of food consumption, GI will show the rise of the blood sugar level. GI does not show the individual's response to different glycemic food. But represents a general increase in the glucose levels in reaction to all the macronutrients taken.

Another important term which is related to glycemic index is the glycemic load. This load is calculated by multiplying the actual serving of the meal with the glycemic index of the food taken. The load is what holds more significance for individuals as it indicates the impact of the sugars. For example, watermelon has a much high glycemic value but low glycemic load because of the small quantity it is taken or consumed. Whereas the fructose has a low glycemic index but high glycemic load due to the amount of the large quantity of the serving.

So, the mere consideration of the values is not enough to categorize food as being good for diabetes or bad. We also need to consider the serving, amount and time of the day while assessing a meal as diabetic friendly or not.

Classification of Food on the Basis of Glycemic Index:

Glycemic index classifies the food items into three broad categories. And these are as follows:

1. **Low GI:**

The low glycemic food has a value of 55 or less. These products are ideal for a diabetic diet and are recommended to everyone who is intolerant to high glucose. the tables in this chapter will give you the idea of low glycemic fruits, vegetables, etc. Not all fruits are low Glycemic, and not all are high. This variation exists throughout every category of the food item.

2. **Medium GI:**

the medium range starts from 56 GI value and ends at 69 GI value. It is not that ideal, but it is safer to stay in this range than moving to the high GI items. Certain fruits and vegetables lie in this category. You can take a small amount of these food items in a day to keep the glucose level maintained.

3. **High GI**

Food is having the GI value 70 or above are in the red zone that the highest range for glycemic index. These items are completely forbidden on a low carb diet. They can cause an immediate hike in the blood glucose level.

Classification	GI range
Low GI	55 or less
Medium GI	56–69
High GI	70 and above

Following is the list of the commonly used food items which are categorized as being low, medium and high glycemic food. This short list is here to give you an idea to compare to grocery list:

Low GI Foods (55 or less):

- 100% stone-ground whole wheat or pumpernickel bread

- Oatmeal (rolled or steel-cut), oat bran, muesli
- Pasta converted rice, barley, bulger
- lima/butter beans, peas, legumes and lentils
- Most fruits, non-starchy vegetables and carrots

Medium GI (56-69):

- Whole wheat, rye, and pita bread
- Quick Oats
- Brown, wild or basmati rice, couscous

High GI (70 or more):

- White bread or bagel
- Cornflakes, puffed rice, bran flakes, instant oatmeal
- Short grain white rice, rice pasta, macaroni and cheese from mix
- Russet potato, pumpkin
- Pretzels, rice cakes, popcorn, saltine crackers
- melons and pineapple

The Meal Plan

Let's get right into the fun! Time to focus on the delicious foods that will be consumed from here on out. The following meal plan combines it all to simplify and ease the transition. Looking forward we have meal plans, recipes, etc. The home kitchen will be your new restaurant as you whip up delicious snacks and meals to lose weight and manage your diabetes.

Week 1

The Primer

We understand that this entire ordeal and journey can be cumbersome and stressful but if you stay dedicated, the fruits of your labor will show! Experimenting with different foods and meals can be daunting however once you try our recipes and the utilize the following sample 7 day meal plan you will understand just how delicious and fun it can actually be. Let's take the unknown out of it all and jump right into some healthy eating.

	Breakfast	Lunch	Dinner	Dessert
Sunday	Bacon Bok Choy	Roasted Cauliflower	Zucchini Mushroom Lasagna	Buckwheat Chocolate Cake
Monday	Bacon Wrapped Egg Muffins	Balsamic Tomato Chicken	Prosciutto Chicken	Chia Coco Pudding
Tuesday	Spinach Morning Muffins	Steak with Caramelized Fennel	Avocado Beef Fajitas	Creamy Chocolate Mousse
Wednesday	Hazelnut Cheese Breakfast	Green Ham Soup	Queso Chicken Chili	Lemon Curd Pie
Thursday	Coco Protein Oats	Spinach Cheese Rolls	Chicken Piccata	Blueberry Almond Tart
Friday	Cheese Oats Pancakes	Turkey Spinach Meatballs	Balsamic Turkey Breast	Meringue Custard Dessert

| Saturday | Pumpkin Cinnamon Pancakes | Chicken Pesto Casserole | Pork Chops in Tomato Gravy | Coconut Bounty Bars |

Bacon Wrapped Egg Muffins

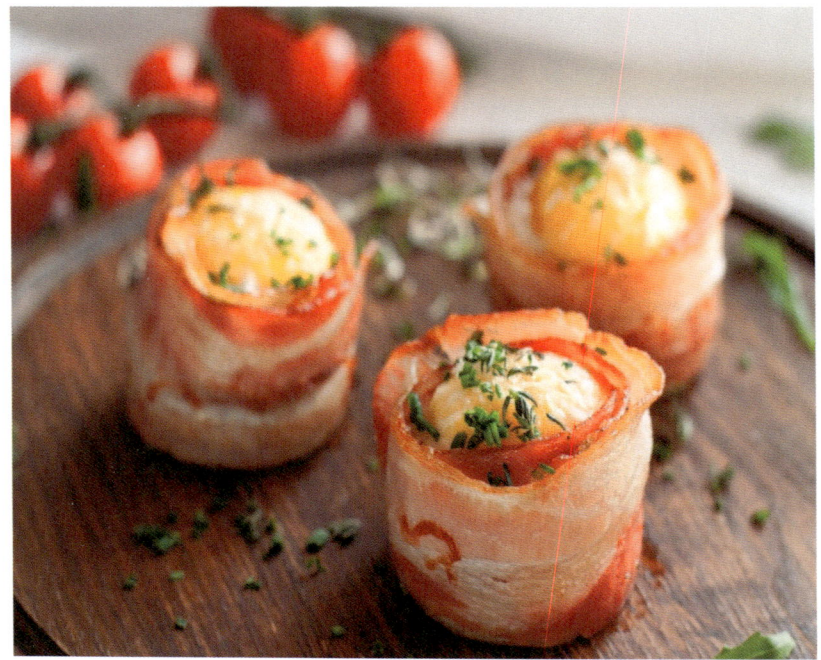

Breakfast Recipes

Bacon Wrapped Egg Muffins

These are low carb egg muffins which are nicely wrapped and baked with turkey bacon slices. These muffins are made out of a rich mixture of eggs with vegetables including bell pepper, jalapeno, garlic, spinach, and onions. Serve these immediately after the bake

Servings: 4

Ingredients

12 slices of **lean turkey bacon**

20 oz. **egg whites**

3 small **eggs**

2½ oz. lean **turkey sausage**

2½ oz. **red bell pepper**

2 oz. baby **spinach**, chopped

3 oz. yellow **onion,** chopped

1 **garlic** clove, minced

½ **Jalapeno Chili,** chopped

1½ teaspoon **salt**

1 teaspoon **pepper**

Directions

Adjust the oven to 350 degrees F.

Spray a muffin tray with cooking spray.

Layer each muffin cup with bacon slices and add spinach at the bottom.

Sauté garlic, onions, and jalapeno in a greased skillet.

Divide this onion mixture into the muffin cups and top with the remaining spinach.

Add sausage and bell pepper on top.

Mix egg whites with pepper, salt, eggs in a bowl.

Pour this egg whites mixture into the muffin cups.

Bake them for 25 minutes.

Serve.

Nutritional Information: 218 calories; 4.3 g fat (0.5 g saturated fat); 60 mg cholesterol; 560 mg sodium; 0.5 g carbohydrates; 0.6 g dietary fiber; 1.3 g total sugars; 10.8g protein.

Blueberry Oat Pancakes

Ditch the same old ordinary pancakes and enjoy a lot more filling and delicious oats pancakes. They are made out of an oatmeal batter and then served with fresh blueberries on top. You can garnish with these any sugar-free topping syrup of your choice.

Servings: 4

Ingredients

½ cup uncooked **oats**

3 **egg whites**

1 scoop vanilla **protein powder**

1 oz. **blueberries**

½ teaspoon **baking powder**

Stevia in the raw, to taste

¼ cup **water**

Cooking spray

Sugar-free syrup (optional)

Directions

Beat everything in a blender except sugar-free syrup and cooking spray.

Layer a skillet with cooking spray and heat it.

Pour a quarter cup of the batter into the skillet and swirl the pan to spread it evenly.

Cook for 1-2 minutes per side.

Make more pancakes then garnish them with sugar-free syrup and berries.

Nutritional Information: 118 calories; 1.8 g fat (0.3 g saturated fat); 5 mg cholesterol; 157 mg sodium; 16.6 g carbohydrates; 2.3 g dietary fiber; 2.4 g total sugars; 22.2g protein.

Salmon Cheese Wraps

To refresh yourself with a protein-rich breakfast, these salmon cheese wraps can be your best shot. The cheesy salmon filling is stuffed inside a low carb tortilla. Such tortillas are made out of almond or coconut flour instead of wheat flour.

Servings: 1

Ingredients

1 8-inch low carb flour **tortilla**

2 oz. smoked **salmon**

2 teaspoon low-fat **cream cheese**

1¼ oz. **red onion**

Handful **arugula**

½ teaspoon fresh or dried **basil**

Pinch of **pepper**

Directions

Heat the tortilla in a microwave for a few seconds.

Mix cream cheese with pepper and basil.

Spread this mixture in tortilla.

Add onion, arugula, and salmon to the tortilla.

Roll them tightly and serve.

Nutritional Information: 241 calories; 15.2 g fat (8.5g saturated fat); 50 mg cholesterol; 112mg sodium; 17.8g carbohydrates; 6.7 g dietary fiber; 3 g total sugars; 23.8g protein.

Hazelnut Cheese Breakfast

Cottage cheese is one healthy choice for all diabetic patients. This cottage cheese blend with crunchy hazelnuts, coconut flakes, blackberries, and pomegranate are great to serve in the morning for a kicking start. Refrigerating well before serving will enhance the taste.

Servings: **2**

Ingredients

½ cup low fat **cottage cheese**

¼ cup **blackberries**

seeds from the ¼ **pomegranate**

½ oz. unsweetened **coconut flakes**

1 oz. **hazelnuts**

Directions

Grind the cottage cheese in a processor until creamy.

Top the cottage cheese with coconut flakes, pomegranate seeds, berries, hazelnuts.

Refrigerate for 2 -3 hours.

Serve.

Nutritional Information: 231 calories; 14.5 g fat (6g saturated fat); 5 mg cholesterol; 387mg sodium; 18.8g carbohydrates; 0 g dietary fiber; 11.6 g total sugars; 17.8 g protein.

Spinach Morning Muffins

All the goodness of eggs, tomatoes, spinach, bacon, cheese, and almond milk is packed inside these mini morning muffins. Its batter is simple to make and easy to store. So, keep it ready in your refrigerator for a quick meal.

Servings: 8

Ingredients

4 cherry **tomatoes**

¼ cup **red onion**, chopped

1 cup **spinach,** chopped

8 **egg yolks**

⅓ cup cooked **bacon**, crumbled

1⅕ cup **cheddar cheese**, shredded

3 tablespoons unsweetened **almond milk** (optional)

½ teaspoon **garlic salt**

Directions

Adjust the oven to 400 degrees F.

Beat egg yolks separately in a bowl.

Add tomatoes, onion, spinach, cheese, almond milk, garlic salt, and bacon.

Pour this egg yolk mixture into muffin tray and drizzle cheese on top.

Bake for 12 minutes.

Serve.

Nutritional Information: 233 calories; 31.6g fat (14.9 g saturated fat); 560mg cholesterol; 360 mg sodium; 5 g carbohydrates; 0.5 g dietary fiber; 1.7g total sugars; 25g protein.

Coco Protein Oats

The tradition of having a nice bowl of oatmeal in the morning is not new. Let's just add a new twist and boosting energy to the same old recipes with some protein and cocoa powder. Make sure to use their unsweetened varieties to cut down the sugars.

Servings: **1**

Ingredients

2 oz. low-fat Greek **yogurt**

0.7 oz. **oats**

½ scoop vanilla **protein powder**

1 teaspoon unsweetened **cocoa powder**

½ cup **almond milk**

Almonds & **berries**

1 teaspoon **Stevia**

Directions

Beat yogurt with cocoa powder, stevia, almond milk, and protein powder.

Pour this mixture into the serving bowl and fold in oats.

Cover the bowl and refrigerate overnight.

Garnish with berries and almonds.

Serve.

Nutritional Information: 243 calories; 3.2 g fat (4.3 g saturated fat); 228 mg cholesterol; 160 mg sodium; 20 g carbohydrates; 0 g dietary fiber; 0.5 g total sugars; 21.4 g protein.

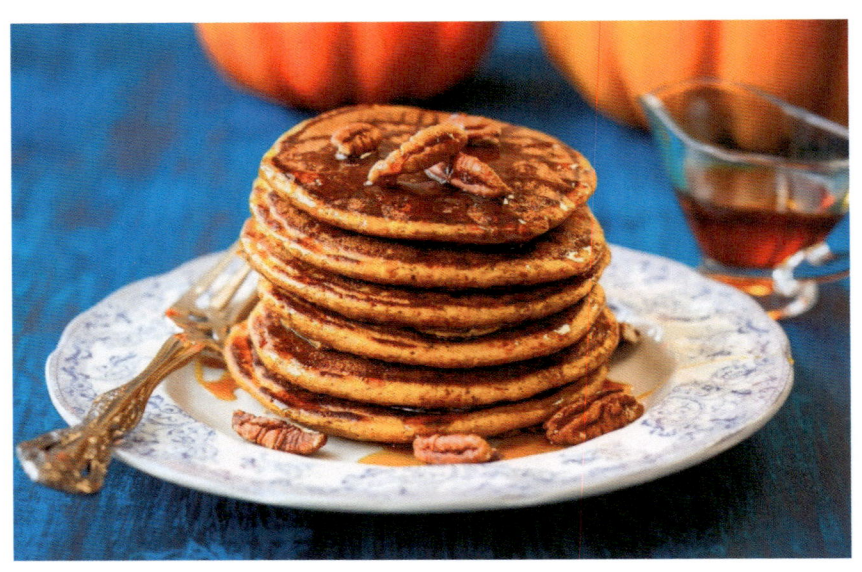

Pumpkin Cinnamon Pancakes

Let's add some pumpkin puree and cinnamon to the basic pancake recipe and enjoy something as delicious as these pumpkin pancakes. Adding stevia for sweetness is completely up to. If you do not have a sweet tooth, then consider it optional.

Servings: 5

Ingredients

0.7 oz. **oats**

3.2 oz. liquid **egg whites**

1 oz. **pumpkin puree**

1 scoop **Vital Proteins**

½ teaspoon **cinnamon**

2 teaspoon **Stevia**

Cooking spray

Apple (optional)

Directions

Blend everything in a blender except cooking spray.

Spray a small pan with cooking spray and heat it.

Pour 1/3 batter into the greased pan and swirl around to spread evenly.

Cook for 2 minutes per side until golden brown.

Use the entire batter to make more pancakes.

Garnish with apple pieces and sugar-free syrup.

Serve.

Nutritional Information: 212 calories; 1.3 g fat (0 g saturated fat); 0 mg cholesterol; 217 mg sodium; 16.5 g carbohydrates; 2.7 g dietary fiber; 1.5 g total sugars; 22.6 g protein.

Cauliflower Meal

It is a perfect substitute to give yourself a break from morning oatmeal. It is similar in texture, but the taste is unique as we will be using cauliflower in it along with peanut butter, cinnamon, almond milk, stevia, and a strawberry. You can add any other berries of your choice.

Servings: 2

Ingredients

1 cup **cauliflower rice**

½ cup unsweetened **almond milk**

½ teaspoon **cinnamon**

¼ teaspoon **Stevia**

½ tablespoon **peanut butter**

1 **strawberry**, sliced

Directions

Add cauliflower rice to a pot of boiling milk along with cinnamon and stevia.

Stir cook for 10 minutes until the milk is reduced.

Garnish with peanut butter and strawberries slices.

Serve.

Nutritional Information: 221 calories; 6.6 g fat (4.3 g saturated fat); 228mg cholesterol; 230 mg sodium; 16.3 g carbohydrates; 7.3 g dietary fiber; 5.8 g total sugars; 6.8 g protein.

Cheese Oats Pancakes

You will fall for the earthy taste of the cottage cheese pancakes. They are so full of calories yet low on carbs. The oats give this meal lots of dietary fibers, which are great when you are suffering from diabetes.

Servings: 4

Ingredients

½ cup low-fat **cottage cheese**

¼ cup **oats**

⅓ cup **Egg Whites**

1 teaspoon **vanilla extract**

1 tablespoon **Stevia** in the raw

Directions

Blend cottage cheese with egg whites, oats, stevia and vanilla extract.

Heat a greased frying pan and add 1/4 of the batter.

Spread it evenly and cook until golden from both the sides.

Garnish with sugar-free jam and berries.

Nutritional Information: 118 calories; 1.5 g fat (0.2 g saturated fat); 5 mg cholesterol; 580 mg sodium; 19 g carbohydrates; 2 g dietary fiber; 5.5 g total sugars; 24.5 g protein.

Bacon Bok Choy

It is basically a bok choy samba, which is a basic mixture of cream with cheese, bok choy, and bacon. The vegetable and bacon are sautéed first and then mixed with all the seasonings and the remaining ingredients.

Servings: **3**

Ingredients:

4 tablespoons **cream**

½ cup **Parmesan cheese**, grated

4 **bok choy**, sliced

2 **bacon** slices

Salt and black pepper, to taste

Directions:

Mix bok choy with salt and black pepper in a bowl and keep it aside.

Heat oil over medium heat in a frying pan and sauté bacon slices for 5 minutes.

Add bok choy and cream to the pan and cook for 6 minutes.

Top the mixture with Parmesan cheese.

Cover it first then cook on low heat for 3 minutes.

Serve warm.

Nutritional Information: 121 calories; 12.5 g fat (0.2 g saturated fat); 5 mg cholesterol; 580 mg sodium; 9 g carbohydrates; 2 g dietary fiber; 1.5 g total sugars; 2.5 g protein.

Balsamic Tomato Chicken

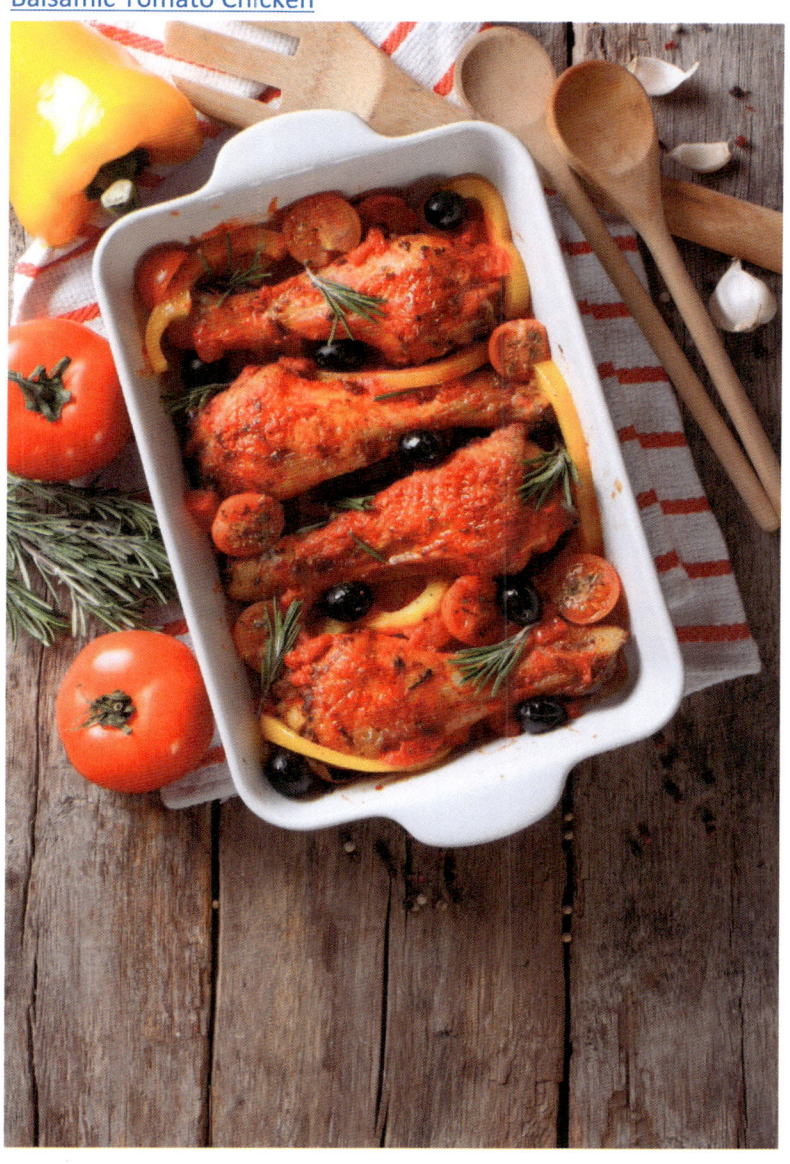

Lunch Recipes

Roasted Cauliflower

Crispy and crunchy cauliflower florets are great to serve as a luncheon when prepared with the special garlic sauce, cheese and tangy spices, used in this recipe. Just bake till the florets turn golden and then enjoy the crisp.

Servings: **6**

Ingredients

6 tablespoons **olive oil**, divided

1 tablespoon **butter**

3 tablespoons chopped **tomato**

2 tablespoons **orange juice**

2 teaspoons minced **chipotle** in adobo

¾ teaspoon kosher **salt**, divided

10 cups **cauliflower** florets

¼ cup crumbled **Cotija cheese**

1 tablespoon chopped fresh **cilantro**

Directions

Adjust your oven to 450 degrees F.

Add butter, garlic, and 4.5 tablespoons oil in a saucepan.

Cook this mixture until it simmers then decrease the heat.

Cook for 20 minutes until garlic is soft.

Allow it to cool then blend along with salt, chipotle, tomato and orange juice.

Toss cauliflower with oil and salt in a baking sheet.

Bake them for 20 minutes then top them with garlic sauce, cilantro, and cheese.

Serve.

Nutritional Information: 168 calories; 13 g fat (3 g saturated fat); 228 mg cholesterol; 324 mg sodium; 10 g carbohydrates; 0 g dietary fiber; 0.5 g total sugars; 4 g protein.

Green Beans with Mushroom Sauce

A dollop of mushroom sauce always tastes amazing in any combination. Here is served with parboiled, seasoned green beans. It has everything rich in its ingredients, from cream to broth, shallots, chives, etc.

Servings: **4**

Ingredients

2 cups sliced **shallots**, divided

6 tablespoons **olive oil**

1 cup sliced cremini **mushrooms**

4 cloves **garlic**, sliced

1 cup heavy **cream**

4 cups **mushroom** broth

2 pounds **green beans**, sliced into 1-inch pieces

½ teaspoon **salt**

2 tablespoons minced fresh **chives**

Directions:

Heat a greased skillet and add 1.5 cup shallots. Sauté for 6 minutes until brown.

Keep the fried shallot in a plate lined with paper towel.

Now sauté mushrooms in the same pan for 2 minutes.

Stir in garlic and shallots. Cook for 1 minute.

Add cream and cook until reduced to halt.

Pour in broth and stir cook for 25 minutes.

Meanwhile, parboil the green beans in boiling water for 3 minutes.

Immediately transfer them to an ice bath.

Puree the mushroom mixture and add it to the drained beans in a pot.

Stir cook for 3 minutes.

Garnish with chives and shallots.

Serve.

Nutritional Information: 214 calories; 17 g fat (7 g saturated fat); 328 mg cholesterol; 317 mg sodium; 13 g carbohydrates; 4 g dietary fiber; 6 g total sugars; 3 g protein.

Oysters with Almond Butter

Oysters sound delicious and healthy. Now you can enjoy them with our delicious anchovy almond butter. Here the oysters are broiled with the butter mixture, and then it served. Garnish with some chopped parsley for more taste.

***Servings:* 12**

Ingredients

24 large **oysters,** scrubbed

4 tablespoons unsalted **butter**, softened

¼ cup skinless **almonds**, finely chopped

3 **anchovy fillets**, minced

1 tablespoon **mayonnaise**

1 tablespoon chopped **parsley**

1 teaspoon grated **orange zest**

Pinch of **cayenne pepper**

Directions

Adjust the broiler to high temperature.

Layer a baking sheet with balls of foil or rock salt.

Prepare the oysters by shucking it and remove the top shells.

Strain them using a fine sieve and reserve the oyster liquid.

Keep the prepared oysters in the pan with their shell side down.

Mix almonds with butter, parsley, anchovies, mayonnaise, cayenne and orange zest in a bowl.

Stir in 1 ½ tablespoon oyster liquor.

Top the oysters with this butter mixture and broil them for 5 minutes.

Serve instantly.

Nutritional Information: 102 calories; 10 g fat (4 g saturated fat); 138 mg cholesterol; 32 mg sodium; 2 g carbohydrates; 0 g dietary fiber; 0 g total sugars; 2 g protein.

Roasted Turnips

There are many ways to enjoy turnips, but this recipe beats every other in taste and aroma as it brings your crispy roasted turnips with special salt and vinegar seasoning. The turnips are first boiled for a while and then roasted with other ingredients.

Servings: 4

Ingredients

1½ pounds **turnips**, peeled and cut into 1-inch wedges

3 cups **water**

½ cup **cider vinegar** plus 1 tablespoon, divided

2 tablespoons **olive oil**

½ teaspoon **salt**, divided

1½ teaspoons chopped fresh **chives**

Directions:

Adjust the oven to 450 degrees F.

Add turnips to boiling water along with ½ cup vinegar.

Decrease the heat and cover the simmering pot.

Cook for 10 minutes then drain the turnips.

Spread the turnips in a baking sheet and bake for 25 minutes.

Toss the roasted turnips with salt, vinegar, and chives.

Serve.

Nutritional Information: 212 calories; 7 g fat (1 g saturated fat); 123 mg cholesterol; 160 mg sodium; 9 g carbohydrates; 2 g dietary fiber; 5 g total sugars; 2 g protein.

Escarole Cream Salad

Having salad in the day is good for the health, especially when you are dealing with diabetes. This recipe provides a good option for all; it is full of fruits like apple, red grapes, and escarole, cream, yogurt, and necessary seasonings.

Servings: **4**

Ingredients

½ cup **walnuts**

3 tablespoons **olive oil**, divided

Pinch of **salt** plus ½ teaspoon, divided

2 tablespoons **sour cream**

2 tablespoons whole-milk plain **yogurt**

1 tablespoon **cider vinegar**

½ teaspoon ground **pepper**

1 medium head **escarole**, torn into ½-inch pieces

1 medium **apple**, thinly sliced

1 cup thinly sliced **celery**

1 cup seedless **red grapes**, halved

Directions

Pulse all the walnuts in a food processor until coarsely ground.

Heat a skillet, greased with 1 tablespoon oil.

Add walnuts with salt. Sauté for 2 minutes.

Keep the walnuts in a plate.

Mix sour cream with pepper, yogurt, vinegar, salt, and 2 tbsp. oil in a bowl.

Stir in celery, grapes, apples, and escarole.

Garnish with roasted walnuts.

Serve.

Nutritional Information: 279 calories; 12 g fat (3 g saturated fat); 321 mg cholesterol; 291 mg sodium; 15 g carbohydrates; 4 g dietary fiber; 0 g total sugars; 4 g protein.

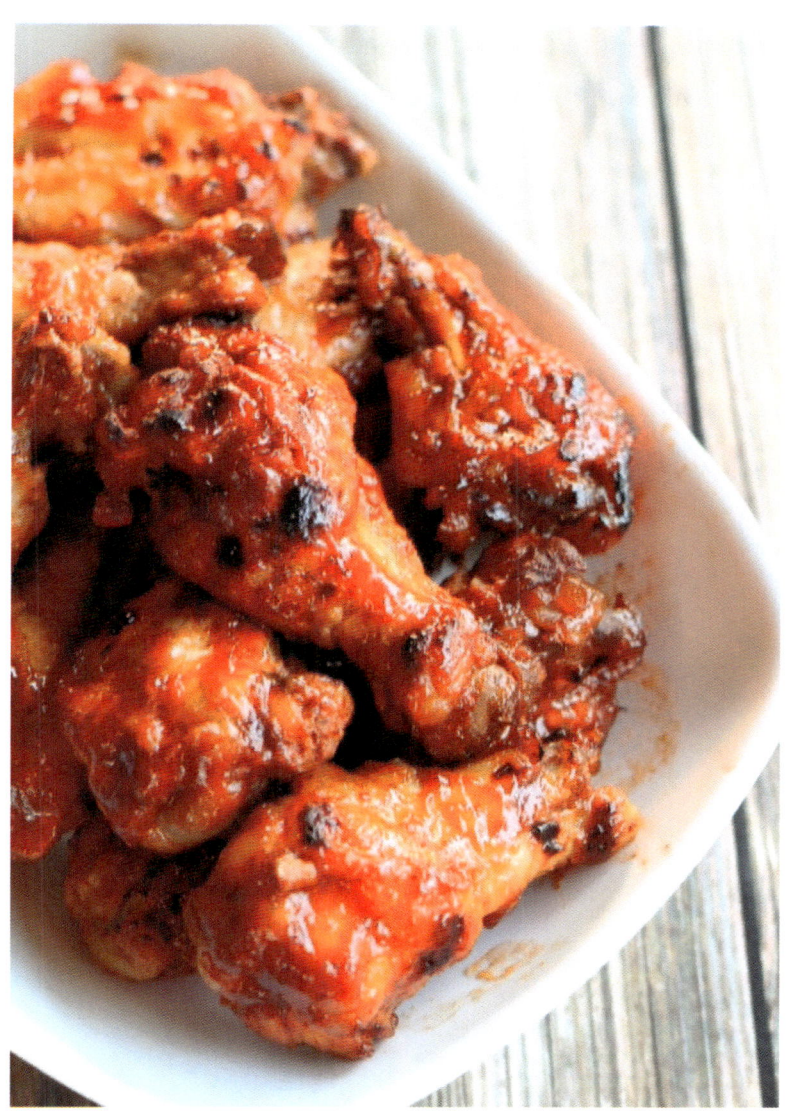

Balsamic Tomato Chicken

You can add some poultry to the menu by using this luscious chicken recipe. Here the chicken is cooked in a special tomato gravy. The magic ingredients of this recipe are the roasted fennel seeds, which add a distinct taste and aroma to the dish.

Servings: 4

Ingredients

2 8-ounce boneless, skinless **chicken breasts**, sliced in 4 pieces

½ teaspoon **salt**, divided

½ teaspoon **ground pepper**, divided

¼ cup white whole-wheat **flour**

3 tablespoons **olive oil**, divided

½ cup halved **cherry tomatoes**

2 tablespoons sliced **shallot**

¼ cup **balsamic vinegar**

1 cup low-sodium **chicken broth**

1 tablespoon minced **garlic**

1 tablespoon **fennel seeds**, toasted and lightly crushed

1 tablespoon **butter**

Directions

Pound the chicken breasts wrapped in plastic, with a mallet.

Sprinkle salt and pepper over the chicken.

Dredge the chicken pieces through flour and shake off the excess.

Add 2 tablespoon oil to a skillet and heat it.

Sauté the chicken pieces for 3 minutes per side.

Keep the sautéed chicken in a plate.

Sauté shallot and tomatoes in the same pan for 3 minutes.

Add vinegar and cook for 45 secs then stir in garlic, broth, salt, pepper and fennel seeds.

Cook for 7 minutes then adds butter.

Pour this sauce over the chicken.

Serve warm.

Nutritional Information: 294 calories; 17 g fat (4 g saturated fat); 311 mg cholesterol; 371 mg sodium; 9 g carbohydrates; 1 g dietary fiber; 3 g total sugars; 25 g protein.

Cholesterol 311 mg

Green Ham Soup

There could be no better way of having broccoli on a diabetic diet than having it in this delicious ham soup. there is not just broccoli but a blend of a number of vegetables including cauliflower, spinach, and onion. Serve with boiled egg and ham on top.

Servings: 4

Ingredients

2 tablespoons **olive oil**, divided

4 ounces thick-cut **ham or prosciutto**, diced

1 small **onion**, chopped

2 cloves **garlic**, minced

4 cups low-sodium **chicken broth**

4 cups **broccoli florets**, chopped

2 cups **cauliflower florets**, chopped

2 teaspoons fresh **thyme** leaves

⅛ teaspoon **salt**

4 cups **baby spinach**

¼ cup **parsley**, chopped

8 cups **water**

2 tablespoons distilled **white vinegar**

4 large **eggs**

Directions

Add a tbsp. oil to a pot and heat it.

Add ham to sauté for 3 minutes then keep it aside in a plate.

Sauté onion in the same pot for 3 minutes then add garlic.

Cook for 1 min and add cauliflower, salt, thyme, broth, and broccoli.

Cook, it covered, for 6 minutes

Stir in parsley and spinach. Let it sit for 5 minutes without heating.

Puree this soup using a handheld blender.

Keep it covered and warm.

Meanwhile, crack an into boiling water and cook for 4 minutes.

Serve the soup with cooked egg, ham and parsley on top.

Nutritional Information: 266 calories; 15 g fat (4 g saturated fat); 145 mg cholesterol; 671 mg sodium; 14 g carbohydrates; 5 g dietary fiber; 0 g total sugars; 22 g protein.

Chicken Cauliflower casserole

Every casserole gives you a culinary experience of a lifetime. This chicken cauliflower is not any lesser than the rest. It has cream, cheese, butter, leek, and tomatoes in combination with chicken and cauliflower.

Servings: **4**

Ingredients:

1 cup **heavy cream**

½ **lemon**, the juice

2 lbs. **chicken thighs**

3 tablespoons **butter**

1 lb. **cauliflower**, diced

1 **leek**, diced

4 oz. **cherry tomatoes**, diced

7 oz. shredded **cheese**

salt and pepper

Directions:

Adjust your oven to 400 degrees F (200°C).

Combine cream with pesto and lemon juice, salt and pepper in a bowl. Set it aside.

Drizzle salt and pepper over the chicken thighs and season them generously.

Heat butter in a skillet and sear the thighs in the butter until golden brown from all the side. Transfer the thighs to a greased baking dish and top them with cream sauce.

Add leeks, tomatoes, cauliflower florets and cheese on top of the chicken.

Bake for 30 minutes in the middles portion of the oven.

Serve warm.

Nutritional Information: 321 calories; 19 g fat (6 g saturated fat); 354 mg cholesterol; 160 mg sodium; 10 g carbohydrates; 4 g dietary fiber; 0 g total sugars; 28 g protein.

Steak with Caramelized Fennel

Let's enjoy some juicy steak on the menu. Add something more to the taste with the complementary caramelized fennel. The combination of seasoning used with both the fennel and the steak makes them even more inspiring and irresistible.

Servings: **4**

Ingredients

2 medium **fennel bulbs** with fronds,

1-pound boneless strip **steak**

1 clove **garlic**, grated

¾ teaspoon **salt**, divided

2 tablespoons extra-virgin **olive oil**

¼ cup red **wine vinegar**

1 tablespoon chopped fresh **sage**

Directions

Chop only half cup fronds and thinly slice the rest.

Slice the steak into ¼ inch cubes.

Toss the steak with garlic and salt in a bowl.

Make ¾ inch thick patties out of the steak mixture.

Sear these patties for 5 minutes per side in a heated, greased pan.

Keep the patties in a plate, aside.

Add fennel slices to the same pan and sauté for 3 minutes.

Stir in salt, sage, and vinegar.

Cook for 5 minutes then add chopped fennel.

Serve the patties with this fennel sauce.

Nutritional Information: 322 calories; 19 g fat (8 g saturated fat); 354 mg cholesterol; 160 mg sodium; 13 g carbohydrates; 3 g dietary fiber; 0 g total sugars; 21 g protein.

Chicken Pesto casserole

If you ever have tried chicken pesto and then this casserole will also make you drool a bit. It makes excellent use of the pesto, whether red or green. Other than chicken, the casserole is loaded with olives, cream, and cheese.

Servings: **4**

Ingredients:

1½ lbs. **chicken thighs** or chicken breasts

2 oz. **butter**, for frying

3 oz. **red pesto** or green pesto

1½ cups heavy whipping **cream**

8 tablespoons pitted **olives**

8 oz. **feta cheese**, diced

1 **garlic** clove, minced

Salt and pepper, to taste

To serve

5 1/3 oz. leafy **greens**

4 tablespoons **olive oil**

sea salt and ground black pepper

Directions:

Adjust the oven to 400 degrees F (200°C).

Dice the chicken into bite-sized pieces. Add salt and pepper.

Melt butter in a large skillet and fry the chicken pieces, in batches, on medium heat until golden in color.

Mix pesto and cream in a glass container.

Place the chicken pieces in a baking pan along with olives, feta cheese, and garlic. Add the pesto.

Bake in oven for 30 minutes, until the dish turns bubbly and light brown around the edges.

Nutritional Information: 351 calories; 9 g fat (6 g saturated fat); 54 mg cholesterol; 760 mg sodium; 18 g carbohydrates; 3.1 g dietary fiber; 1 g total sugars; 38 g protein.

Zucchini Mushroom Lasagna

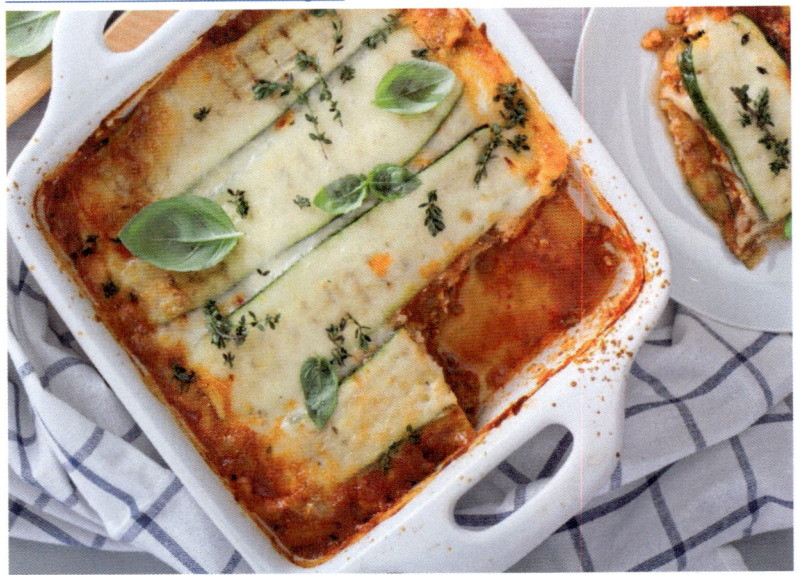

Dinner Recipes

Zucchini Mushroom Lasagna

We all love lasagna, and no health-oriented diet should avoid us having a piece of that, that is why we bring you a rich and delicious zucchini mushrooms lasagna. It has everything healthy whether it's the nutritious vegetables or shredded mozzarella.

Servings: 4

Ingredients

16 oz. **ground beef**, 92%

2 medium **zucchinis**, sliced

4½ oz. **onion**, chopped

2 cloves **garlic**, chopped

1 **serrano chili**, chopped

3 **tomatoes**, sliced

5½ oz. **mushrooms**, chopped

½ cube **chicken bouillon**

½ cup shredded low-fat **mozzarella**

1 teaspoon **paprika**

1 teaspoon dried **thyme**

1 teaspoon dried **basil**

Salt & pepper

Cooking spray

Directions

Keep the sliced zucchini in a colander and sprinkle salt on it.

Let it sit and drain for 10 minutes then pat dry the slices with a paper towel.

Broil the zucchini for 3 minutes in the oven at high heat.

Again, dry it using a paper towel.

Carve an X on top of each tomato and add them to boiling water for 3 minutes approximately.

Transfer them instantly to an ice bath then peel off the skin.

Chop tomatoes along with other vegetables.

Sauté onion, garlic, and chili in a greased pan for 1 minute.

Stir in mushrooms and tomatoes. Sauté for 4 minutes.

Add beef, spices, and paprika. Cook until beef turns brown.

Add chicken bouillon and cook for 25 minutes on low heat.

Meanwhile, adjust oven to 375 degrees F.

Spread a parchment sheet in a baking tray and spread 1/3 zucchini at the base.

Add a layer of meat sauce on top of zucchini.

Now spread 1/3 zucchini over the meat sauce.

Repeat the layer until meat sauce and zucchini are completely used.

Top the lasagna with cheese and bake for 35 minutes.

Slice and serve.

Nutritional Information: 311 calories; 7.9 g fat (3.5 g saturated fat); 67.5mg cholesterol; 558 mg sodium; 12.3 g carbohydrates; 3.6 g dietary fiber; 6.3 g total sugars; 30.4 g protein.

Spinach Cheese Rolls

Rolls may not sound suitable for a dinner meal, but these are no ordinary rolls, these are made out of layers of cheese and spinach. They provide a good number of calories along with all the necessary macronutrients. Enjoy them with some cauliflower rice for the best experience.

Servings: **4**

Ingredients

16 oz. **spinach** leaves

3 **eggs**

2½ oz. **onion**, chopped

2 oz. **carrot**, grated

1 oz. low-fat **mozzarella** cheese

4 oz. fat-free **cottage cheese**

¾ cup **parsley**, chopped

1 cloves **garlic,** chopped

1 teaspoon **curry** powder

¼ teaspoon **chili** flakes

1 teaspoon **salt**

1 teaspoon **pepper**

Cooking spray

Directions

Adjust the oven to 400 degrees F.

Mix spinach with garlic, salt, pepper, 2 eggs and mozzarella in a bowl.

Spread a parchment sheet in a baking tray and oil it with cooking spray.

Add spinach mixture and spread into 10x12 inch rectangle.

Bake it for 15 minutes then allow it to cool.

Sauté onion in a pan greased with cooking spray.

Add parsley and carrots. Sauté for 2 minutes.

Stir in cottage cheese, salt, pepper and curry chili.

Remove the cottage cheese mixture from the heat and add an egg.

Mix well and spread it over the baked spinach sheet while leaving the corners.

Roll the spinach sheet carefully and bake again for 25 minutes.

Slice and serve.

Nutritional Information: 276 calories; 10.4 g fat (4.6 g saturated fat); 326 mg cholesterol; 695 mg sodium; 19.6 g carbohydrates; 5.1 g dietary fiber; 6.7 g total sugars; 27.3 g protein.

White Chicken Soup

It is basically a coconut milk soup, which has chicken in a combination of different vegetables including juicy zucchini and cubed pumpkins. Bell pepper adds quite a strong flavor to the soup. Serve it with warm garlic bread slices.

Servings: 4

Ingredients

1 lb. **chicken breast**, thinly sliced

Salt & pepper, to taste

1 tablespoon **coconut oil**

1 small **onion**, sliced

2 **garlic** cloves, minced

1-inch piece **ginger**, peeled and minced

1 medium **zucchini**, diced

1 cup **pumpkin,** cubed

1 **red bell pepper**, thinly sliced

1 small **chili or jalapeño pepper**, thinly sliced

14 oz. **coconut milk**

2 cups **chicken broth**

Juice of 1 **lime**

Handful **cilantro** leaves

Directions

Add salt and pepper to the chicken breast to season it well.

Take a pot soup and heat coconut oil in it.

Add seasoned chicken and sauté for 5 minutes.

Stir in ginger, garlic, and onion. Stir cook for 3 minutes.

Add pumpkin, zucchini, bell pepper, coconut milk, broth, lime juice, and chili or jalapeno.

Stir cook to a boil then let it simmer on low heat for 20 minutes.

Garnish with cilantro.

Serve.

Nutritional Information: 263 calories; 12.7 g fat (5.5 g saturated fat); 3.7 mg cholesterol; 753 mg sodium; 11.6 g carbohydrates; 1.7 g dietary fiber; 5 g total sugars; 17.1 g protein.

Balsamic Turkey Breast

When you plan to have poultry in a day, turkey breast is another good option, considering the taste and the texture. This meal is also good for all the festive occasion. The turkey breast is marinated in balsamic vinegar marinade which infuses a unique flavor into it.

Servings: 2

Ingredients

- 1 lb. **turkey breast**, diced
- 1 teaspoon **olive oil**
- 1½ teaspoon **balsamic vinegar**
- ¼ teaspoon **garlic powder**
- ¼ teaspoon dried **basil**
- ¼ teaspoon **thyme**
- ¼ teaspoon **pepper**

Directions

Mix thyme, pepper, vinegar, garlic powder, olive oil and basil in a Ziploc bag.

Add turkey breast chunks to the bag and seal it.

Refrigerate for 30 minutes for marination.

Sear the marinated turkey for 8 minutes in a greased skillet until al dente.

Serve warm.

Nutritional Information: 284 calories; 13.5 g fat (1.8 g saturated fat); 110 mg cholesterol; 171 mg sodium; 4.6 g carbohydrates; 0.7 g dietary fiber; 2.2 g total sugars; 41.3 g protein.

Avocado Beef Fajitas

The idea of serving beef fajitas at the dinner table will excite you. It is a mixture of fresh peppers and the beef strips. All the ingredients are sautéed in the basic spices along with line juice. It can be served with low carb tortilla or warm bread.

Servings: **2**

Ingredients

1 lb. **beef** stir-fry strips

1 medium **red onion**

1 **red bell pepper**

1 **yellow bell pepper**

½ teaspoon **cumin**

½ teaspoon **chili powder**

splash of **oil**

Salt

Pepper

Juice of half a **lime**

Freshly chopped **coriander**

1 **avocado**

Directions

Take an iron skillet and heat it with a splash of oil.

Slice the bell peppers into ¼ inch thick slices.

Sear the beef strips for 1 minute per side in the hot skillet.

Sprinkle salt and pepper for seasoning.

Keep these stripes aside in a plate.

Add bell peppers and onion to the same pan and sauté with cumin and chili powder.

Sauté for 5 minutes.

Add lemon juice, avocado, and coriander.

Serve.

Nutritional Information: 283 calories; 16.8 g fat (5.2 g saturated fat); 86 mg cholesterol; 67 mg sodium; 10.5 g carbohydrates; 4.4 g dietary fiber; 1.2 g total sugars; 30 g protein.

Prosciutto Chicken

The chicken breast in this recipe is wrapped in sliced prosciutto and then baked with cream cheese, basil leaves and pepper. The chicken is sliced after the baking. You can serve it with your favorite sauce and a refreshing bowl of salad.

Servings: **1**

Ingredients

1 **chicken breast**

1.4 oz. finely sliced **prosciutto**

1.3 oz. **cream cheese**

5-10 fresh **basil leaves**

Pepper

Directions

Spread the prosciutto slices on an aluminum sheet while slightly overlapping their edges.

Top the slices with a layer of cream cheese.

Sprinkle basil leaves and pepper on top.

Place the chicken breast at the center of the prosciutto slices.

Start rolling them around the chicken.

Bake the wrap for 25 minutes at 380 degrees F.

Slice and serve.

Nutritional Information: 263 calories; 11.5 g fat (7.8 g saturated fat); 241 mg cholesterol; 934 mg sodium; 241 g carbohydrates; 0 g dietary fiber; 2.4 g total sugars; 38.6 g protein.

Pork Chops in Tomato Gravy

this saucy pork chops recipe brings you an inspiring combination of seared chops with tomato gravy. This is not it, the gravy is seasoned with dried herbs and served with shredded cheese on top. Make sure to season the chops well while searing.

Servings: 4

Ingredients

4 Thick **pork chops**

1 small yellow **onion**

4 cloves **garlic**

28 oz. diced canned **tomatoes**

5 oz. low-fat **mozzarella**

1 Knorr chicken **bouillon cube**

1 teaspoon **paprika**

1 teaspoon dried **oregano**

Salt & pepper

Cooking spray

Directions

Adjust your oven to 400 degrees F.

Layer a cooking pan with cooking spray.

Sear the pork chops for 2 mins per side. Sprinkle salt and pepper.

Transfer the chops to a baking dish.

Add garlic and onion rings to the same pan. Sauté for 1 minute.

Add spices, tomato and bouillon cubes.

Cook for 2 minutes then pours this mixture over pork chops.

Drizzle cheese on top and bake for 20 min.

Serve.

Nutritional Information: 237 calories; 17.1 g fat (8 g saturated fat); 114 mg cholesterol; 160 mg sodium; 16.2 g carbohydrates; 1.3 g dietary fiber; 3.4 g total sugars; 43.5g protein.

Queso Chicken Chili

It is time to put your Instant Pot to better use and make this delicious chicken chili recipe. The chicken is cooked in salsa Verde along with garlic, onion, oregano, and cumin. Once cooked it is topped with queso fresco, avocados, radish for best taste.

Servings: 6

Ingredients

1 tablespoon **vegetable oil**

1 yellow **onion**, diced

4 cloves **garlic**, minced

1 teaspoon ground **cumin**

1 teaspoon **oregano**

2½ lbs. **chicken breasts**, boneless & skinless

16 oz. **salsa Verde**

Toppings

2 packages **queso fresco**, crumbled

2 **avocados**, diced

8 **radishes,** chopped fine

8 sprigs **cilantro** (optional)

Direction

Adjust the Instant Pot to the sauté setting on medium heat.

Add vegetable oil and onion. Sauté for 3 mins at maximum.

Stir in garlic and saute more for 1 minute.

Now add oregano, cumin, and ½ of the salsa.

Keep the chicken breasts at the base of the Instant Pot and top them with remaining salsa.

Seal the Pot lid and set it for 10 minutes on manual function.

Once done, release the pressure naturally.

Shred the chicken into fine pieces and return it to the pot.

Serve warm.

Nutritional Information: 261 calories; 12.3 g fat (2.3 g saturated fat); 71.9 mg cholesterol; 542 mg sodium; 9.1 g carbohydrates; 3.8 g dietary fiber; 3.3 g total sugars; 30.1 g protein.

Turkey Spinach Meatballs

These meatballs can be taken directly with any sauce, or you can add them to zucchini noodles or try them with some cauliflower rice or boiled brown rice. The use of oats in the recipe makes these meatballs equally soft and crunchy.

***Servings:* 4**

Ingredients

20 oz. ground **turkey**

4 oz. fresh or frozen **spinach**

¼ cup **oats**

2 **egg whites**

2 **celery sticks**, chopped

3 cloves **garlic**, chopped

½ green **bell pepper**, chopped

½ red **onion**, chopped

½ cup **parsley**, chopped

½ teaspoon **cumin**

1 teaspoon **mustard** powder

1 teaspoon **thyme**

½ teaspoon **turmeric**

½ teaspoon **chipotle** pepper

1 teaspoon **salt**

Pinch of **pepper**

Directions

Adjust the oven to 350 F (175 C)

Mix all the vegetables with turkey, oats, spices and egg whites in a bowl.

Layer a baking tray with parchment paper.

Make meatballs out of this mixture.

Place them in the baking tray and bake for 25 minutes.

Serve warm.

Nutritional Information: 253 calories; 2.5 g fat (0.6 g saturated fat); 55.3 mg cholesterol; 582 mg sodium; 12 g carbohydrates; 3.1 g dietary fiber; 2.9 g total sugars; 31 g protein.

Chicken Piccata

If you haven't yet tried chicken piccata then here is a recipe which you can try even on a diabetic diet. it is made out of chicken breasts, butter, white wine, stock, capers, and parsley. All these ingredients are cooked in a saucy base with a little seasoning on the side.

Servings: 4

Ingredients

2 skinless, boneless **chicken breasts**, sliced

3 tablespoon unsalted **butter**

1½ tablespoon all-purpose **flour**

¼ teaspoon **white pepper**

¼ teaspoon **salt**

2 tablespoon **olive oil**

⅓ cup dry **white wine**

⅓ cup low sodium **chicken stock**

¼ cup **lemon juice**

¼ cup drained **capers**

¼ cup Italian **Parsley** minced

Salt & pepper

Directions

Pound the chicken slices into ½ inch thickness using a mallet.

Season flour with pepper and salt in a shallow dish.

Dredge the chicken slices through the flour and shake off the excess.

Heat a greased sauté pan and sear the chicken slices for 4 minutes per side.

Stir in wine, lemon juice, and stock. Cook for 3 minutes until it thickens.

Add butter, parsley, and capers.

Serve.

Nutritional Information: 244 calories; 15.7 g fat (6.6 g saturated fat); 72.6 mg cholesterol; 457mg sodium; 3.4 g carbohydrates; 0.6 g dietary fiber; 0.4 g total sugars; 20.3 g protein.

[Peanut Butter Chocolate Brownie](#)

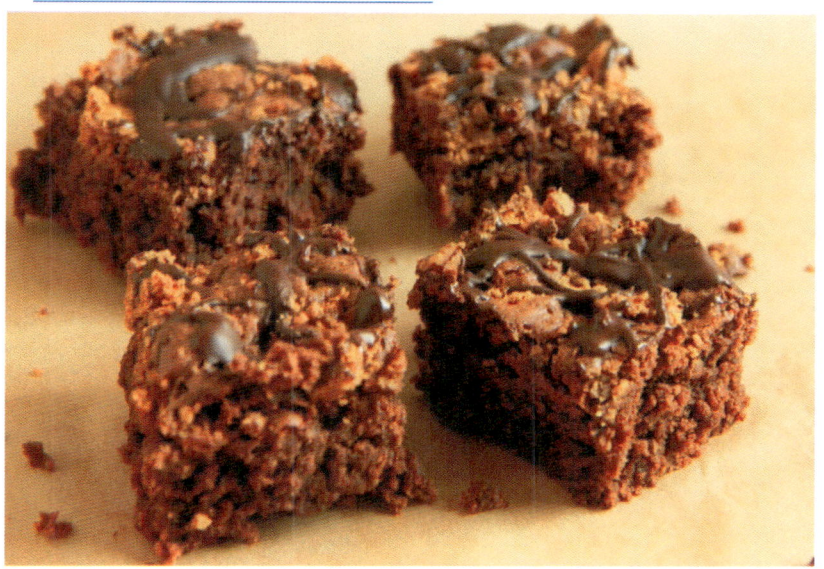

Dessert Recipes

Buckwheat Chocolate Cake

Diabetic diet won't stop you from enjoying some soft and fluffy cake. Here is the recipe which is completely sugar-free, yet it is equally delicious. It is prepared out of buckwheat flour; you can also use almond flour or coconut flour.

Servings: **6**

Ingredients

7 oz unsweetened 100 % dark **chocolate**

2 tablespoons **butter**

4 whole **eggs**

1 egg **yolk**

Swerve, to taste

1 oz **cornflour**

1 oz **buckwheat** flour

1/4 cup **coconut milk**

Directions

Adjust the oven to 360 degrees F. Grease four ramekin with oil.

Heat chocolate with butter in a saucepan until it melts. Keep it aside.

Whisk eggs with sweetener and egg yolk in a mixer.

Stir in buckwheat flour and corn flour. Mix until smooth.

Heat coconut milk in a saucepan then pours it into egg mixture with continuous stirring.

Add in chocolate melts then divide the batter into the ramekins.

Bake for 15 minutes.

Serve.

Nutritional Information: 148 calories; 4.7 g fat (2.3 g saturated fat); 176 mg cholesterol; 36 mg sodium; 12.5 g carbohydrates; 0.5 g dietary fiber; 4.5 g total sugars; 1.4 g protein.

Meringue Custard dessert

this dessert recipe is a combination of lightly prepared vanilla custard and poached meringue. First, the custard is prepared using coconut milk and vanilla extract and then it is topped with egg meringue, almonds, and raspberries.

Servings: **2**

Ingredients

Vanilla custard

2 cup canned **coconut milk**

1 teaspoon **vanilla extract**

4 **egg yolk**

1 cup **swerve** sweetener

Poached Meringue

4 **egg white**

2 tablespoons **swerve**

Garnish

2 tablespoons sliced **almonds**

1/4 cup **raspberries** fresh or defrost

Directions

Vanilla Custard

Heat milk mixed with vanilla in a saucepan until it boils.

Separate egg yolk from egg whites.

Beat egg yolk with sugar-free sweetener in an electric mixer until fluffy.

Pour in lukewarm vanilla milk and mix well.

Heat the combined mixture in a saucepan and cook for 10 minutes on low heat until it thickens.

Refrigerate the custard until further used.

Prepare the meringue

Beat egg white with sweetener in an electric mixer until foamy.

Boil 1-liter water in a saucepan and add egg white mixture scoop by scoop.

Let it poach for 30 seconds on both sides.

Serve the custard with meringue, melted chocolate, caramel, almonds, and raspberries.

Nutritional Information: 274 calories; 0.7 g fat (2.1 g saturated fat); 31 mg cholesterol; 21 mg sodium; 22.5 g carbohydrates; 0.3 g dietary fiber; 4.5 g total sugars; 0.4 g protein.

Avocado Brownies

You will certainly enjoy having a chocolate brownie with the twist of inspiring avocado flavor. The recipe is simple; its batter is prepared out of almond meal, eggs, avocado flesh, and chocolate bites. Some baking soda will make the brownies softer and spongier.

Servings: 4

Ingredients

3 oz unsweetened dark **chocolate** bites

2 teaspoons virgin **coconut oil**

1 cup ripe **avocado** flesh

2 **eggs**

1/2 cup **erythritol**

1/2 cup **almond meal**

1/2 cup unsweetened **cocoa powder**

1/2 teaspoon **baking soda**

1/4 teaspoon **salt**

1 teaspoon **vanilla extract**

Directions

Adjust the oven to 350F. Layer a 24x24 cm brownie pan with a parchment sheet.

Melt chocolate bites with coconut oil in a saucepan.

Blend avocado flesh, almond meal, eggs, erythritol, cocoa powder, salt, baking soda, vanilla extract and melted chocolate in a blender.

Pour the avocado batter into the square pan. Spread it evenly.

Bake for 30 minutes.

Cool and slice the brownies.

Serve.

Nutritional Information: 265 calories; 0.6 g fat (1.2 g saturated fat); 145 mg cholesterol; 311 mg sodium; 15.5 g carbohydrates; 0.3 g dietary fiber; 3.2 g total sugars; 0.4 g protein.

Lemon Curd Pie

this pie is made out of coconut flour crust and stuffed with lemon curd pie filling. It is prepared out egg yolk, eggs, lemon juice, and a sweetener. This pie has to be served once it is cooled, after refrigerator for 2 hours at least. Slice and enjoy.

Servings: **6**

Ingredients

1 coconut flour pie **crust** dough

1/2 cup **lemon juice**

2 **eggs**

2 **egg yolk**

1/2 cup **coconut oil**

1/4 cup **erythritol**

2 **egg white**

Directions

Beat egg yolks with eggs, lemon juice and sweetener in a saucepan.

Heat this mixture then add coconut oil with occasional stirring.

Increase the heat and cook until it all thickens.

Remove the egg yolks mixture from the heat then allow to cool for 15 minutes.

Spread the crust in a pie pan and fill with its lemon curd.

Refrigerate for 2 hours.

Serve

Nutritional Information: 138 calories; 2.7 g fat (4.1 g saturated fat); 22 mg cholesterol; 43 mg sodium; 11.5 g carbohydrates; 0.4 g dietary fiber; 2.3 g total sugars; 1.6 g protein.

Peanut Butter Chocolate Brownie

Every dessert menu is almost incomplete without some brownie. This chocolate brownie is prepared using peanut butter, cocoa powder, almond milk, and almond meal. It is one mug microwave recipe which takes a minute to bake.

***Servings:* 1**

Ingredients

2 tablespoon **almond meal**

2 tablespoon **almond milk**

1 tablespoon crunchy **peanut butter**

1 tablespoon unsweetened **cocoa powder**

1 teaspoon **erythritol powder**

or 1/4 teaspoon **stevia powder**

1 teaspoon sugar-free **chocolate chips**

Directions

Mix almond flour with sweetener, milk and cocoa powder in a mug.

Stir in peanut butter and chocolate chips.

Microwave it for 40 seconds on high heat.

Serve immediately.

Nutritional Information: 218 calories; 3.3 g fat (1.3 g saturated fat); 21 mg cholesterol; 34 mg sodium; 19.5 g carbohydrates; 0 g dietary fiber; 0.5 g total sugars; 7.4 g protein.

Roasted Cashew Cookies

These cashew cookies are great to serve as an after-meal dessert or as a snack. These cookies are prepared out of coconut flour, chocolate chips, coconut, and roasted cashews. Avoid overbaking the cookies; else they will lose their essential moisture and the texture.

Servings: 4

Ingredients

2 cup unsweetened **desiccated coconut**

2 tablespoon **coconut flour**

3/4 cup **cashews nut**, roasted

¼ cup extra virgin **coconut oil**, melted

2 **eggs**

1/4 cup sugar-free **chocolate chips**

1/4 cup **Swerve**

1 tablespoon **vanilla extract**

Directions

Adjust the oven 320 degrees F.

Layer a cookie sheet with a parchment sheet. Keep it aside.

Blend everything in a blender leaving just chocolate chips.

Fold in chocolate chips and make 8 cookies out of this dough.

Place the cookies in the cookie sheet and bake for 20 minutes.

Serve

Nutritional Information: 211 calories; 1.7 g fat (4.5 g saturated fat); 212 mg cholesterol; 53 mg sodium; 17.5 g carbohydrates; 0.6 g dietary fiber; 0.5 g total sugars; 6.1 g protein.

Creamy Chocolate mousse

It is one simple mousse recipe. The coconut cream is mixed with beaten egg whites and cocoa powder. The mousse is then refrigerated for some time. Garnish the mousse either with sugar-free chocolate chips, or sliced strawberries or blueberries.

Servings: **2**

Ingredients

3 **egg whites**

1 cup **coconut cream** full cream canned

4 tablespoon unsweetened **cocoa powder**

2 tablespoons **swerve**

Directions

Separate egg yolks from egg whites.

Beat egg whites in an electric mixer for 2 minutes.

Add xylitol and mix well.

Slow stir in coconut cream, and cocoa powder.

Refrigerate the mousse for 2 hours.

Garnish with coconut flakes.

Serve.

Nutritional Information: 121 calories; 1.5 g fat (1.2 g saturated fat); 322 mg cholesterol; 143 mg sodium; 12.5 g carbohydrates; 0 g dietary fiber; 0.5 g total sugars; 7.4 g protein.

Coconut Bounty Bars

Here is a quick and easy bounty bars recipe. The sweet bar is stuffed with coconut and coconut cream stuffing and coated with a layer of chocolate on the outside. Use sugar-free chocolate for the coating.

Servings: 4

Ingredients

2 cups unsweetened desiccated **coconut**

1/2 cup **coconut cream** canned

1/3 cup **erythritol**

1/3 cup extra virgin **coconut oil**

Chocolate coating

6 oz sugar-free **chocolate chips**

2 teaspoon extra virgin **coconut oil**

1-2 **stevia** drops -to taste

Directions

Layer a 10 inches square pan with a plastic wrap.

Blend everything in a blender except chocolate coating.

Mix well until the dough is smooth.

Wrap the dough with the plastic wrap and freeze for 10 minutes.

Cut the dough into 20 bars.

Melt chocolate chips with stevia drops in the microwave by heating for 30 secs.

Dip each bar into the chocolate melt.

Freeze the bars for 10 minutes.

Serve.

Nutritional Information: 281 calories; 9.7 g fat (4.3 g saturated fat); 228 mg cholesterol; 160 mg sodium; 0.5 g carbohydrates; 0 g dietary fiber; 0.5 g total sugars; 7.4 g protein.

Blueberry Almond Tart

Here is a sweet and savory almond tart recipe which is filled with blueberry stuffing and topped with almond walnut crust. Add chia seeds to the filling makes it all more delicious and healthier. Always serve fresh.

Servings: 4

Ingredients

Walnuts Almond Crust

1 cup **walnuts**

6 tablespoon **almond meal**

2 tablespoon **coconut oil**

1 **egg white**

Vanilla extract 2-3 drops

Filling

1 cup frozen **blueberries**

2 tablespoon **chia seeds**

Directions

Walnuts Almond Crust

Grind everything in a food processor and turn the dough into a ball.

Wrap this ball with a plastic wrap and roll it into a crust.

Place this almond crust in the pie mound.

Filling

Mix chia seeds with blueberries in a bowl.

Pour this mixture into the crust.

Make a criss-cross design on top using some remaining dough crust.

Bake for 25 minutes.

Serve.

Nutritional Information: 221 calories; 0.7 g fat (1.3 g saturated fat); 28 mg cholesterol; 16 mg sodium; 21.5 g carbohydrates; 0 g dietary fiber; 3.2 g total sugars; 0.4 g protein.

Chia Coco Pudding

If you are up for a bowl of pudding, then chia coco pudding is one great option. It is prepared out of chia seeds, cocoa powder, and almond milk. Stevia is used for sweetening of the pudding whereas you can also use Swerve. Garnish with your favorite topping.

Servings: 2

Ingredients

1/3 cup **Chia Seeds**

1/4 cup. unsweetened **cocoa powder**

Stevia, to taste

1/3 cup **Raw Cacao** (Nibs)

2 1/2 cup Sugar-free Chocolate **Almond Milk**

Directions

Mix chia seeds, stevia, cocoa nibs, cocoa powder and milk in a bowl.

Cover chia seeds mixture and put it in the refrigerator for 4 hours.

Garnish with cocoa nibs, berries, and coconut cream.

Serve.

Nutritional Information: 253 calories; 10.2 g fat (5.3 g saturated fat); 312 mg cholesterol; 11 mg sodium; 17.5 g carbohydrates; 0.4 g dietary fiber; 12.5 g total sugars; 0.4 g protein.

Conclusion:

Dealing with diabetes as a health condition is not easy, it takes time to comprehend the gravity of the problem. But with the right approach and correct knowledge, you can easily maintain the blood glucose levels without entirely depending on the medications and possibly even reversing the type 2 diabetes. This cookbook can take you one step closer to that approach. It has discussed diabetes at length and suggested the ways to control and prevent the harms of this diseases. The section for the recipe shares some of the delicious ways to enjoy all the natural flavors without any fear of a hike in sugar levels.

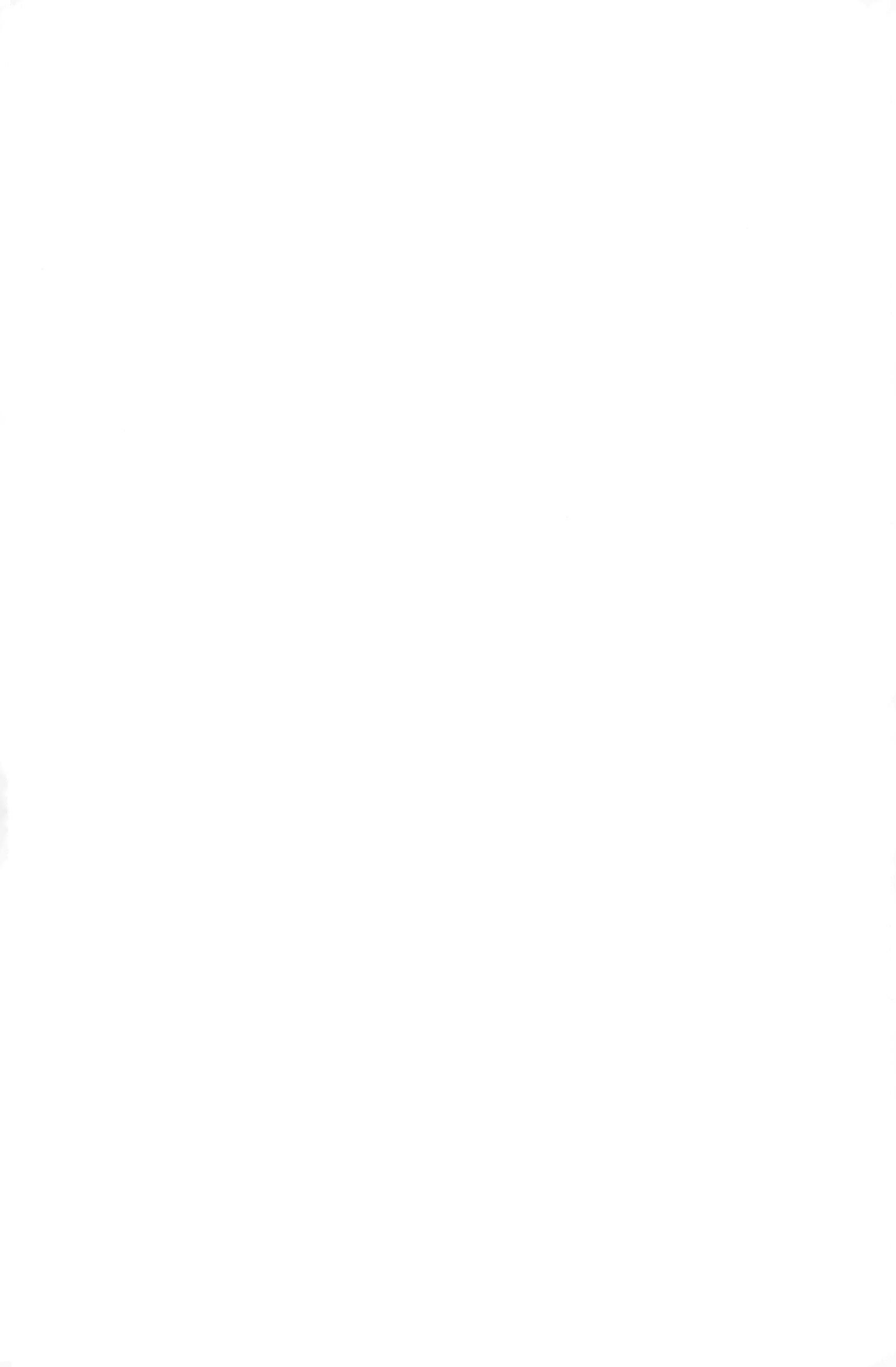

Printed in Great Britain
by Amazon